Awakening Your Inner Warrior

Secrets to Unshakeable Confidence

Table of Contents

Each of us must confront our own fears, must come face to face with them. How we handle our fears will determine where we go with the rest of our lives. To experience adventure or to be limited by the fear of it.

— Judy Blume

Chapter 1. Introduction

Unleash the limitless potential buzzing within you, waiting to be released, with our Special Report: "Awakening Your Inner Warrior: Secrets to Unshakeable Confidence." This comprehensive guide dives headfirst into the realm of personal development and transformation, providing you with the keys to acknowledge and embrace your strengths while banishing fears and doubts. Bursting with actionable insights and powerful techniques, the report will let you tap into your fierce warrior spirit, equipping you not just to survive but triumph in any activity, endeavor, or challenge that life throws at you. With our special report by your side, get ready to unravel the inherent confidence you've always harbored but couldn't quite touch. Now is your time. Light up the path to self-discovery, unveil your true greatness, and walk proudly upon the exciting journey towards an unshakeably confident you. Infuse your life with the vigor of a warrior, start this transformative ride today!

Chapter 2. Discovering Your Inner Warrior: An Introduction

Before we embark on this journey of self-discovery and realization, it is essential to grasp the essence of the warrior spirit. Picture yourself, not merely as a human being, wandering the landscape of life aimlessly, but instead as a seasoned and fearless warrior, who possesses both the will and the capability to take control of their existence, despite the ups and downs awaiting us. The warrior within you encapsulates this ideology to its fullest, serving as a beacon of unshakeable confidence and unwavering resilience.

2.1. Unearthing the Ideals of the Inner Warrior

The very notion of an inner warrior might have struck you as an exotic, distant concept. However, our inner warrior lies not in a faraway realm but infuses the core of our being. Unknowingly, we have been standing atop the treasure chest of this immense might, oblivious to its existence within us. This wellspring of strength and resilience remains untapped for the most part, yet is a reservoir of potential teetering on the edge of revelation. Striking the surface is the first mission on our quest to awaken our powerful warrior within.

When we say 'warrior,' your mind might default to envisioning an armored knight or a martial arts expert. But the essence of the inner warrior transcends the boundaries imposed by these physical representations. A warrior brims with internal qualities: unfaltering courage, enduring tenacity, invincible willpower, humility, and, above all, an unshakeable self-belief that empowers them to navigate their life journey with purpose and conviction even in the face of adversity.

2.2. Defining the Warrior Within: A Deeper Grasp

The warrior within is the embodiment of your deepest strengths and potential. It represents your ability to face challenges with a clear mind, a firm spirit, and an unwavering belief in yourself. The inner warrior is your ally in the journey of life, guiding you towards your goals with unshakeable resilience and confidence.

The inherent warrior within us is a symbol of our unwavering resolve, our courage to stand tall against adversities, our tenacity to stay relentless in our pursuit, and our strength to rise victorious against any pressure. Being a warrior doesn't necessarily connote battling others, shattering bodies and breaking bones. More often than not, it implies winning battles within ourselves – confronting our fears, insecurities, self-doubt, and hesitation. This quest to awaken your inner warrior is much more about befriending and strengthening oneself than combating external forces.

From banishing fears to embracing challenges, unlocking potential to harnessing energy, each aspect of awaking this inner warrior is crucial. By cultivating resilience, building disciplined persistence, thriving under stressful situations, and sustaining this unshakable confidence, the warrior spirit emerges, takes charge, and propels you towards the life you envision.

2.3. Embracing the Journey: The Invocation of Your Inner Warrior

Invoking this power is not as simple as uttering an incantation. Awakening your inner warrior requires conscious effort, boundless resilience, and an enduring belief in your innate capabilities. This quest to unlock the potential is a journey, not a destination. It unwinds through a series of steps, each posing a challenge, each providing a lesson, and each paving the way towards the ultimate goal of self-discovery and empowerment.

As we navigate through this journey together, understand that the process of awakening your warrior spirit is individualised. There's no set route or map; instead, there are merely guidelines and tactics, each aligning with diverse personalities and realms of life. Your process will be as unique as you are, customized to match your experiences, ambitions, and innate strengths.

Unleashing this hidden force within is not about becoming somebody else but rather intensifying who you already are. It's about recognizing your inherent potentials, honing them, and using them as your sword and shield in the relentless pursuit of personal growth and success.

In the subsequent chapters, we will delve further into the intricacies of this process. We will navigate the paths to unlocking your potential, banishing self-doubt, embracing challenges, harnessing inner energy, cultivating resilience, embracing the warrior spirit, instilling discipline, displaying courage under fire, and finally, living as a warrior. These subsequent chapters aim to arm you with the knowledge, strategies, and exercises needed to awaken and nurture the mighty warrior within you.

Gear up to embark on this remarkable journey of self-discovery and self-empowerment. Let the pursuit of awakening the warrior within begin!

Chapter 3. Unlocking Your Potential: The Power of Self-Belief

In this guide, we delve into the primal essence of self-belief—that life-altering, innate conviction you carry about your abilities, purpose and worth. As we embark on this journey of self-discovery, we will uncover the power of self-belief and how it shapes our potential.

3.1. The Essence of Self-Belief

Self-belief is the confidence in one's own abilities, the quiet assurance that propels you to chase your aspirations no matter the odds. It's like possessing a personal catalyst, an inner motor that energizes and propels you forward regardless of external conditions. Self-belief is understanding your potential; it is trusting your judgements, relying on your abilities, and being comfortable with who you are.

With self-belief, the world appears more navigable. Challenges tend not to intimidate you; they only invigorate you. The potency of this quality cannot be underestimated—it's a prerequisite for unlocking your innate potential and exploring the breadth and depth of your capabilities.

3.2. The Physiology of Belief

Our beliefs, including our self-belief, are not simply subjective. They lead to palpable physiological changes, deeply affecting our brain. Studies highlight that positive beliefs help stimulate the growth of new neurons and generate new neuronal connections, which aids in increasing brain capacity. This neurological transformation amplifies your cognitive abilities, such as problem-solving, creativity, and decision-making, thereby enhancing your performance across various life spheres.

On the other hand, harboring negative beliefs can trigger stress responses in the brain, leading to an increased production of cortisol. This "stress hormone" can adversely affect your brain's ability to function optimally, dampening your creative and cognitive potentials. Thus, it becomes apparent that the power of self-belief has far-reaching implications, affecting you on multiple levels, from influencing your brain function to shaping your life.

3.3. The Genesis of Self-Belief

Our self-belief is a amalgamation of experiences, internal dialogues, and the narratives we absorb from our environment. It forms initially during childhood through interactions with our primary caregivers, teachers, and peers. Children who receive consistent encouragement, positive feedback, and emotional support tend to develop a strong sense of self-efficacy, sowing the seeds of robust self-belief.

By the same token, experiences in adulthood also significantly shape our self-belief. From the triumph of conquering a challenging project at work to the resilience shown during a personal crisis, each experience refines our perception of our abilities. Thus, self-belief is not stagnant; it's dynamic and moldable, making personal transformation a real possibility at any life stage.

3.4. Cultivating Self-Belief

Developing self-belief requires deliberate, consistent effort. It begins by acknowledging your unique strengths and qualities, followed by setting realistic goals to prove your capabilities to yourself.

1. *Self-awareness:* This is the bedrock of self-belief. Invest time to reflect on your strengths, weaknesses, values, and ideals. Journaling can be a powerful tool for enhancing self-awareness and tracking growth.

2. *Positive affirmations:* Positive statements about oneself counteract negativity and bolster self-esteem. Daily affirmations reinforce your sense of worth, feeding your self-belief.

3. *Mastery Experiences:* Engage in tasks that challenge you just enough to test your abilities. Successfully navigating these challenges reinforces your self-belief.

4. *Constructive feedback:* Seek feedback from trustworthy sources. Understand that feedback is not a criticism of your worth, but a tool for personal development.

3.5. Overcoming Barriers to Self-Belief

Despite our best intentions, we often face barriers in building self-belief. These barriers can be internal (like self-doubt, fear, or perfectionism) or external (like criticism, failure, or unsupportive environments). Recognizing and overcoming these barriers paves the way for nurturing unwavering self-belief.

1. *Thought Restructuring:* Identifying and altering negative thought patterns helps overcome internal barriers to self-belief. Cognitive-behavioral techniques can be invaluable tools for this transformation.

2. *Resilience Building:* Learning to adapt and bounce back from adversities aids in combatting external roadblocks. Techniques like mindfulness, stress management, and emotional regulation bolster resilience.

3. *Social Support:* Surrounding yourself with a supportive network provides reinforcement and encouragement, reinforcing your

self-belief in the face of external barriers.

In conclusion, self-belief isn't a mere feel-good mantra—it has the power to transform us from within, reshaping our brains, boosting performance, and setting us on the path to realize our unexplored potential. By cultivating self-awareness, embracing positive affirmations, striving for mastery experiences, seeking constructive feedback, and overcoming barriers, we can unlock the power of self-belief, thereby initiating an empowering journey of flourishing and fulfillment.

Chapter 4. Banishing Self-Doubt: The Path to Productive Confidence

In the pursuit of exuding confidence, the first step on the path is to address and banish self-doubt. Self-doubt is like a leech that saps its host of vitality, leaving behind a shell of negative thoughts and feelings. It's essential, therefore, to understand our self-doubt, locate its roots within our psyche, and finally, find ways to shake it off. Let's take a comprehensive journey through the excursion of casting away self-doubt to make room for productive confidence.

4.1. Unpacking the Concept of Self-Doubt

Self-doubt is a psychological state that displays itself as a lack of confidence in one's abilities, talents, and potential. It breeds a crippling fear of failure and can stifle potential, hindering us from even trying to achieve our goals and dreams. Often, this insidious doubt operates in the background like a computer virus, subtly disrupting our thought processes and decision-making abilities. It can manifest in different forms, from overthinking and procrastination to excessive worry about the outcomes of our actions.

4.2. Tracing the Roots of Self-Doubt

Self-doubt rarely emerges out of thin air. Instead, it is the product of our social conditioning, past experiences, and inherited beliefs. Factors such as societal expectations, critical parents, negative feedback, and the constant comparison with others contribute significantly to the formation of self-doubt.

Our brains are naturally skewed towards negative bias – that is, they tend to focus on negative experiences more than positive ones. This negativity bias can reinforce feelings of self-doubt, as our minds continue reminiscing the moments of failure or disappointment while discounting our achievements.

4.3. The Paralysis of Self-Doubt

The effects of self-doubt are pervasive and far-reaching. When we doubt ourselves, we're likely to withhold our ideas for fear of criticism, avoid tasks that push our comfort zones, and procrastinate on important tasks due to fear of a negative outcome.

Self-doubt essentially results in self-censorship, as we restrain ourselves from exploring new ideas, endeavors, and potentials. It curtails creativity and promotes conformity by making the individual skeptical of their unique qualities and abilities.

4.4. Shattering the Shackles of Self-Doubt

The path to banishing self-doubt and fostering productive confidence is paved with self-awareness, self-acceptance, and the cultivation of self-efficacy. Self-awareness helps us to identify our self-doubt triggers, while self-acceptance motivates us to embrace our imperfections and vulnerabilities without judgment.

Cultivating self-efficacy is an essential step to regain confidence in our skills and abilities. Self-efficacy refers to the belief in our capability to execute behaviors required to produce specific outcomes. It encompasses our notions about our competency rather than the actual level of competency. Building self-efficacy empowers us to overcome the paralysis imposed by self-doubt and propels us on the path towards productive confidence.

4.5. Implementing Techniques to Overcome Self-Doubt

There are various strategies available to break the cycle of self-doubt. Affirmative self-talk is one powerful technique that can counter the negative self-perceptions fostering self-doubt. Consistent practice of mindfulness also helps by bringing our attention to the present moment, minimizing the habit of overthinking that often amplifies self-doubt.

Creating a 'Success Log,' where we jot down our daily accomplishments, however small they might be, also greatly assists in nurturing a healthy self-image. Over time, visual evidence of our capabilities strengthens our belief in ourselves and assists in eliminating self-doubt.

4.6. Building Momentum Towards Productive Confidence

Initiating the journey away from self-doubt and towards productive confidence is not a one-time endeavor. It requires consistent practice, patience, and more importantly, compassion towards yourself. Remember, everyone has moments of self-doubt, but it doesn't define you or your worth.

The key lies in not letting self-doubt take the driver's seat. Instead, acknowledge it, accommodate it, and then slowly start to reshape it. As you do so, you pave the way for productive confidence to take root and grow, transforming you into the unshakeable warrior you are meant to be.

Ending this chapter, let it be known that by vigilantly debunking the myths you've told yourself and taking mindful steps towards deep self-acceptance, you can banish self-doubt. As you clear your internal landscape of fears, you reveal a path that is primed for the emergence of fruitful, productive confidence. Remember, the unshakeable confidence of an inner warrior is not a destination, but an exciting and ever-evolving journey.

Chapter 5. Embracing Challenges: How to Grow Amidst Various Obstacles

Stepping into the world of challenges can feel like traversing an uncharted landscape, filled with towering mountains and teeming seas. Many people view these challenges as imposing insurmountable obstacles blocking their path towards bliss. However, the key to self-growth lies in the reconsideration and reframing of these challenges as opportunities for growth. In fact, these challenges are not barricades but bridges, leading us to the fortress of unshakeable confidence and personal development. It is through a deeper understanding of challenges and cultivating the right mindset to accept these challenges, an individual lays the foundation for substantial growth and progress.

5.1. Embracing Challenges as Opportunities

Challenges, big and small, are an inevitable part of life. Instead of dreading them, we must remember that these trials are often disguised opportunities. They push us to think differently, act differently, and come out of our comfort zones, unlocking our true potential. Each challenge presents a lesson, a key that opens the door to profound wisdom and insight. The act of facing a challenge head-on, confronting it, wrestling with it, and overcoming it, changes us significantly. It shapes us into more robust, resilient beings, ready to face the world with courage and conviction.

5.2. Overcoming the Fear of Failure

One of the biggest impediments to embracing challenges is the fear of failure. Often, it is our own self-doubt that limits us, forming invisible chains that keep us from stepping onto the field. The way to shatter these chains is through the acceptance of failure as an integral part of the learning process. Embrace the fact that you will fall, but each fall is another chance to stand up even stronger. It's essential to realize that failure does not define us, rather how we respond to failure indeed does. Taking these lessons to heart, we find that "failure" isn't a foe but rather a strict teacher who guides us towards growth.

5.3. Building a Growth Mindset

The cultivation of a growth mindset is the cornerstone in harnessing the potential to learn from challenges. A growth mindset means viewing intelligence, talent, and skill as a product of dedication and hard work, rather than fixed traits we are born with. Embrace the idea that you can always learn, grow, and improve. Stand on the precipice of challenge with open arms, ready to learn and grow. In this way, each challenge becomes a step forward on our journey of self-discovery and empowerment.

5.4. Cognitive Reframing

Another technique to cultivate a positive outlook towards challenges involves cognitive reframing or cognitive restructuring. This involves changing our perspective of difficulties from stumbling blocks to stepping stones. Change your "I can't" to "I can," and see how the skies open up. Reinvent your narrative and turn it from one of fear to one of courage and determination.

5.5. Resilience and Perseverance

Closely tied to the process of embracing challenges is the cultivation of resilience and perseverance. Resilience is the ability to bounce back from adversity, maintaining your integrity and strength in the face of trials. Perseverance, on the other hand, is the ability to keep going, pushing forward, even when progress seems agonizingly slow and the road becomes rocky. Together, resilience and perseverance form a formidable duo against any challenge, ushering you to your end goals shining in high spirits.

As we journey through life, challenges will come our way one after another. But, by understanding the nature of challenges, overcoming our fear of failure, nurturing a growth mindset, practicing cognitive reframing, and fostering resilience and perseverance, we can strive to invite these challenges into our lives. Embrace them for the opportunities they offer, for they are the ones who bring out the warrior within us, pushing us towards the realm of unshakeable confidence, growth, and personal transformation. So embrace these challenges, for they are the sculptors of the unshakeable inner warrior that resides within each one of us.

Chapter 6. Harnessing your Inner Energy: Maximizing Personal Power

The journey of mastering self-confidence is incomplete without understanding and tapping into the source of it all - your inner energy. This intangible yet highly potent part of you is continuously humming with power waiting to be capitalized on. To maximize personal power, it's essential to create conditions conducive to awakening and channeling your energy in rewarding ways. In this chapter, we'll delve into methods for tapping into your core energy and directing it towards transformative purposes.

6.1. Decoding Inner Energy

Before harnessing this inner energy, an understanding of the concept is indispensable. Inner energy, as the name suggests, emanates from within, influencing everything from your physical strength to your mental resilience. It's the molecular-level vigor that fuels your capacity for creativity, problem-solving, and continuous self-improvement. Reigning in this energy means steering your thoughts, actions, and decisions towards desired outcomes.

The first step is self-awareness, which involves deep introspection and honest self-assessment. Recognize the emotions, passions, and mental stimuli that act as the energy sources for you. Anything that stirs you positively or negatively, provides strength, or evokes passion contributes to your internal energy reservoir.

6.2. Activating Inner Energy

Once identified, the next step is to stir up this latent energy. You can activate your inner energy through several ways, from changes in daily routines to exercises in mindfulness.

Physical exercise acts as a potent energy stimulant. Activities like Tai Chi or Qigong, running, swimming, or dancing invigorate the body, thereby revving up your inner energy. Other activities like yoga and meditation provide a more subtle channel, aligning your physical and mental states to set your energy flow on a steady course.

Mental stimuli like reading a powerful book or engaging in a riveting conversation can also activate your internal energy. These activities excite the mind, causing a surge in your overall energy.

6.3. Channeling Inner Energy for Maximizing Personal Power

Activated energy is great; directed energy is far more potent. In the true spirit of a warrior, it is not just about awakening the energy but channeling it towards productive and transformative causes. Directed inner energy lends strength to your convictions, amplifies your abilities, and drives you towards your goals with unshakeable resolve.

When you learn to focus this energy on a specific task, you'll notice improvements in your productivity and efficiency. It could be something as simple as undertaking your daily tasks or as significant as taking a giant leap towards your dreams and goals. This is where techniques like visualization and goal setting come in, helping to guide your inner energy towards the desired trajectory.

6.4. Tools and Techniques

Monotonous chores and tasks can be transformed into meaningful engagements by applying energy effectively. Here's a detailed rundown on how to direct your energy into areas of importance:

1. Visualization: This involves painting a vivid mental picture of your goal or desired outcome. This technique fires up your energy, aligning it with the goal in mind.

2. Affirmations: Positive self-talk or affirmations steer your energy towards confidence and self-belief. Consistently reminding yourself of your capabilities and strengths helps direct your energy towards significant tasks.

3. Goal-setting: Clear, defined goals act as conduits for your inner energy. With a focused objective, your energy finds a well-charted course to flow through.

4. Mindfulness: Being present in the moment, devoid of past regrets or future anxieties, ensures your energy is applied entirely to the here and now.

6.5. Balancing Energy

It's equally important to maintain a balance in the flow of your inner energy. Overexertion or misdirection of this energy could lead to burnout or ineffective usage. Rest, adequate sleep, and leisure are as critical as consistent work to balance your inner energy, thereby replenishing and revitalizing it.

6.6. Cultivating Habits to Sustain Energy Flow

Finally, make it a point to cultivate habits that help keep your energy levels high. These practices, such as maintaining a balanced diet, getting regular exercise, and making time for relaxation and recreation, will ensure your reserves of inner energy remain constant.

Harnessing your inner energy is an ongoing process. Undertaken with consistency and dedication, it promises to amplify your inner strength, arming you with the resilience, poise, and unwavering belief essential for a warrior navigating the battlefield of life. Pledge yourself to this path, and you will soon witness your personal power climb to new and dizzying heights, a testament to your blooming warrior spirit.

Chapter 7. Cultivating Resilience: Bouncing Back from Difficulties

The journey to self-discovery and empowerment isn't always a smooth sail. More often than not, it is riddled with various forms of adversity that, if mishandled, can erode your zeal and stall your growth. This chapter is a comprehensive guide that not only helps you understand the essence of resilience but also charts a detailed roadmap to effectively and efficiently cultivate it. Resilience is the indefatigable spirit, the ever-burning flame within you that allows you to bounce back from any setback, transforming all your trials into stepping stones towards achieving the goal of unshakeable confidence.

7.1. The Essence of Resilience

Resilience can be understood as a combination of personal attributes, mindsets, and skills that allow an individual to navigate through difficulties and adversities in a healthy and effective manner. But resilience is not the mere ability to resist adversity or escape unharmed. It involves gaining strength, growth, and wisdom from the adversities faced, thereby preparing for future contingencies. The warrior spirit within you has an inherent quality of resilience, but it is the careful nurturing and honing of this characteristic that leads to the unwavering confidence that defines a true warrior.

7.2. Cultivating Personal Traits for Resilience

Certain personal characteristics act as catalysts in attaining and enhancing resilience. They form a part of your internal environment that can be controlled and optimized. Traits like optimism, faith, patience, goal-orientation, emotional stability and understanding your purpose are crucial for fostering resilience. Investing time in self-reflection, introspection, and emotional intelligence exercises can help in cultivating these traits. Adopt practices like mindfulness and meditation that can improve emotional stability and fortify your mental strength to face hardships with resilience.

7.3. Developing Coping Mechanisms

Equally important to fostering resilience are reliable coping mechanisms. Coping mechanisms are strategies that help mitigate the stress induced by challenging situations. Each person's coping mechanism is uniquely individual and largely dependent on their personal traits, experiences, and circumstances. Using healthy coping strategies like stress management, time management, using humor as a coping tool, or seeking support from loved ones can significantly improve your resilience.

7.4. Navigating Through Challenges

Life is a marathon, with myriads of obstacles on the path to your goals. It is important to embrace this reality and foresee challenges as part of life's journey. This preemptive approach will not let adversities catch you by surprise, reducing their impact. Moreover, it is important to identify the lessons embedded in these challenges. Each adversity is an opportunity to learn a new lesson, gain a new skill, and prepare yourself for future challenges.

7.5. Promoting Physical Well-being

While resilience is largely centered on mental strength, physical well-being plays an equally crucial role. Regular exercise, adequate rest, and a balanced diet ensure that your body is equipped to bear the brunt of adversities. Exercise, in particular, can increase the production of stress-relieving and mood-enhancing hormones that can provide the much-needed respite amidst challenging times.

7.6. Fostering a Supportive Social Network

While the journey towards unshakeable confidence is deeply personal, it cannot be undertaken in isolation. The saying "no man is an island" holds an undeniable truth. It is crucial to surround yourself with a supportive network of loved ones who not only provide emotional sustenance but can also give you a different perspective during challenging times. Their support and encouragement play a critical role in maintaining and enhancing resilience.

The journey to becoming your inner warrior is not about reaching a destination but about enjoying and learning from the journey itself. Cultivating resilience is like honing your inner compass, guiding your ship through the stormy seas towards your quest for unshakeable confidence. By nurturing resilience within you, you are not only preparing to face adversities, but also building the bedrock for future growth and unshakeable confidence. One must remember, a resilient warrior is a successful warrior, and a resilient you is an unshakeably confident you. Keep striving, keep learning and remember, every fall is an opportunity to rise stronger, every mistake an opportunity to learn, and every adversity an opportunity to grow.

Chapter 8. The Warrior Spirit: Rising Above Fear and Negativity

All of us encounter various forms of fear and negativity in our everyday lives. It is intrinsic to the human experience. Some endure the fear of failure, the anxiety of rejection, or the uncertainty of change, whereas others grapple with negativity, doubt, and self-criticism. Regardless of the form these mental monsters take, they have the potential to erode our confidence and shackle our potential. However, when you awaken your inner warrior spirit, you can triumph over these intruders decisively.

8.1. Understanding Fear and Negativity

To triumph over fear and negativity, we must first comprehend their nature and how they operate within us. Fear is an emotional response to a perceived threat, and negativity is generally an attitude of pessimism or disbelief in the positive or constructive aspects of life. While they can serve a protective purpose, for example, fear can warn us against immediate danger, and negativity can prevent complacency, they often overstep their boundaries, keeping us trapped in unhelpful behavioral patterns. Continual fear can lead to anxiety, while constant negativity can lead to a depressive state.

We must realize that fear and negativity are created within us, and they pertain more to our perspective on events rather than the events themselves. This nuance can dramatically shift our perspective towards these emotional responses, creating an agency for us to control and work with them productively.

8.2. Awakening the Warrior Within

Once we have educated ourselves about fear and negativity, it's time to awaken the warrior within us. The inner warrior is a metaphorical concept, personifying the courage, strength, resilience, and determination inherent within each of us. Significantly, your inner warrior is not a new entity to be created; instead, it's an innate power waiting to be awakened and utilized.

Influential psychologist Carl Jung referred to this as the "shadow" side of our personality, consisting of latent parts of our psyche that we often reject or ignore. Embracing this shadow side allows us to tap into our power and confront the fears and negativity that hinder our growth. Thus, awakening your inner warrior is essential for rising above fear and negativity.

8.3. Techniques to Harness the Warrior Spirit

To awaken and consistently employ your warrior spirit, certain techniques and practices can prove to be beneficial. These approaches are aimed at strengthening your mental fortitude, instilling a can-do attitude, and creating a stable platform for success even in the face of fear and negativity.

1. Mindfulness and Meditation: These practices help you develop an objective understanding of your fear and negative thoughts. With mindfulness, you observe your thoughts and feelings without judgment, fostering self-awareness. Regular meditation practice can reduce anxieties and negative thought patterns, thereby making room for positive, assertive thoughts.

2. Affirmations: Positive, empowering statements repeated daily can transform your belief system. Saying things like "I am brave," "I am powerful," or "I overcome my fears" can replace the

negative chatter in your mind. When said with conviction and consistency, affirmations can significantly boost your morale and confidence.

3. Physical Exercise: Engaging in physical activities like martial arts, running, or yoga can help in building physical strength and endurance, which naturally translates into mental strength. Remember, a healthy body promotes a healthy mind.

4. Mantaining a Gratitude Journal: Documenting things you are thankful for can help shift your focus from negativity to the numerous sources of positivity and joy around you. This can significantly diminish the impact of negative thoughts and foster an attitude of positivity.

8.4. Squaring off Against Fear and Negativity

Once you have awoken your warrior spirit and have handy techniques at your disposal, it's time to take on fear and negativity head-on. Remember, the goal is not always to eliminate these feelings; that can be an unrealistic expectation given their rootedness in our basic human instincts. Instead, we aim to manage and rise above them.

When you are beset by fear, try to understand what message it's sending you. Is it warning against an imminent threat, or is it arising from an overly cautious mindset? In the face of negativity, challenge your thoughts. Are they valid, or are they being overly critical? Harness the power of your inner warrior to throw light upon these thoughts and combat them effectively.

8.5. Living Above Fear and Negativity: The Warrior Spirit

In sum, the warrior spirit is not devoid of fear or negativity. Instead, it is about understanding, confronting, and managing these feelings. Furthermore, it is the process of enhancing your inherent capabilities and overall self-confidence that allows you to thrive even amidst adversity.

In this process of growth, there will be setbacks and failures, but the warrior spirit within you will ensure that you bounce back each time, stronger than before. Empowering the warrior spirit within you is equivalent to giving yourself the competence not just to survive but to triumph in any environment, circumstance, or challenge that life presents you.

Indeed, the process of continuously rising above fear and negativity embodies the true warrior spirit – it is the essence of an indomitable will, relentless courage, uncompromising resilience, and the unstoppable drive for success. Unleash this force within you, and let your warrior spirit shine amidst the battles of life, conquering fear and negativity with unshakeable confidence.

In conclusion, the path of the warrior is not an easy one. It demands discipline, patience, and commitment, but the rewards are boundless. With the warrior spirit guiding you, the dark clouds of fear and negativity will no longer hinder your journey. Instead, they'll serve as reminders of your resolve, strength, and the conviction that you are indeed, above them all.

Chapter 9. Warrior's Discipline: Building Persistence for Success

In our journey thus far, we've delved deep into the world of the inner warrior, and now we stand at the foot of one of the most central and pivotal concepts in building unshakeable confidence: discipline. discipline is the gritstone upon which we polish the rough edges of our potential, and the steadfast peg that keeps our warrior spirit tethered when storms of fear and doubt rage on. In this extensive exploration of the warrior's discipline, we'll dissect its importance, strategies to cultivate it, and how you can leverage it to build an unwavering resolve for success.

9.1. The Crucial Role of Discipline: Cementing the Path to Success

In the raw, chaotic world we inhabit, discipline serves as the bedrock of orderliness and the compass guiding us through the uncertain terrains of life. For the warrior, discipline is not a mere tool for survival; instead, it is the firm foundation that supports the structure of their habits, efforts, and actions, the nurturing framework that allows their true potential to bloom.

Without discipline, potential remains just potential - undirected and unfulfilled. Discipline is that vital bridge between intending to do something and actually doing it. It transforms the abstract ideal of success into a measurable, tangible outcome derived from consistent actions focused towards that goal. As someone embarking on the mission to awaken their inner warrior, developing and adhering to discipline is paramount in your journey toward success.

9.2. Strategies for Cultivating Discipline: From Seed to Fruit

Cultivating discipline is akin to growing a tree: it requires patience, consistent care, and the ability to bounce back from hosile conditions.

Understand You Can Shape Your Discipline

Firstly, you need to believe that discipline is malleable - not a cemented attribute but a quality you can purposely influence and shape.

Set Clear, Realistic Goals

Next, set clear, realistic goals for yourself rather than ambiguous or far-too-grand aspirational achievements. Having a clear, achievable goal fosters discipline as it gives your efforts a defined objective.

Practice Mindfulness

Mindfulness inculcates discipline. By focusing on the present, you reduce distractions, highlight your actions in relation to your goals, and transition from impulsive to thoughtful, disciplined behavior.

Engage in Regular Exercise and Healthy Diet

A disciplined body fosters a disciplined mind. Regular exercise and a balanced diet strengthen resistance to physical and mental stresses, thereby bolstering a disciplined lifestyle.

9.3. Discipline and Persistence: The Twin Guardians of Success

Discipline reigns not in isolation, but hand in hand with its twin trait, persistence. It conveys us across life's sprawling ocean on the vessel of organized, meaningful effort, while persistence empowers us to tread against the rampaging currents of defeat and despair.

Persistence is that unwavering commitment to keep going when the road seems rugged and unending, when the burdens feels heavy, when failure seems a more ravaging reality than success. It is the courageous voice that whispers to soldier on, when everything else screams to stop. Arming oneself with a resilience that is as tenacious as the primal instinct for survival is crucial for manifesting the astounding portrayal of success.

9.4. Discipline, Persistence, and You: The Winning Trinity

As you embark on this pathway of discipline and persistence, the transformation will not be easy. There will be temptations to deviate and doubts to separate you from your path, but this is where your discipline-supported perseverance should shine brightest.

To master the art of discipline and persistence, internalize their power, apply them in your daily routine, and assess the changes they bring about. Gradually, the thin veil of impossibility will part, replaced by the path of triumph. In turn, this disciplined persistence will ignite transformation and push you one step closer to becoming an unshakeable warrior.

Remember, success is no more than the sum of consistent actions guided by a disciplined focus. It is not an overnight phenomenon but rather the long-term result of your willingness to remain firm when times get tough, remain steadfast when results aren't immediately visible, and persist with an unyielding resolve. With discipline and persistence at your helm, arrive at the shores of success, rested yet resilient, prepared to harness new challenges and carve new victories. Embody the warrior spirit. Forge your legacy with the unwavering flame of discipline and persistence.

Chapter 10. Courage under Fire: Thriving in High-Pressure Situations

Learning to thrive in high-pressure situations may feel like a gargantuan task. However, with the right mindset, tools, and strategies, you can not only survive but flourish in environments that others might find overwhelming or crippling. By honing your agility and resilience, learning to control your emotional response, and using pressure as a catalyst for personal growth and excellence, you can evolve into the epitomic warrior, braving every storm that life pitches at you.

10.1. Understanding High-Pressure Situations

High-pressure situations are stress-inducing scenarios that often arise unexpectedly. They may stem from any sphere of life, be it professional confrontations, family dynamics, personal crises, or societal pressures. The critical thing to remember is, these situations do not demand perfection but require presence, action, and astute decision-making, even when the going gets tough.

10.2. Building Resistance Towards Pressure

Developing resistance towards pressure begins with understanding your stress triggers and finding ways to diffuse them. Practices such as meditation, deep breathing, and mindfulness can help cultivate resilience by calming the mind, enhancing focus, and grounding you in the present moment. Regularly incorporating these practices into your routine transforms the way you perceive and react to stressful situations, thereby reducing their impact on your mental well-being and overall performance.

10.3. Emotional Control in High-Pressure Situations

Emotions play a big role in how you handle high-pressure situations. It's essential to manage your emotional reactivity, as unchecked emotional responses can exacerbate stress, clouding clear judgment and effective decision-making. Cultivating emotional intelligence allows you to recognize, understand, and manage your emotions, paving the path towards more balanced and composed reactions.

Techniques such as cognitive reappraisal, where you reframe your perspective towards stressful events, and self-soothing, where you use comforting measures to calm down, can greatly assist in emotional control.

10.4. Pressure as a Stepping Stone

Intense situations, when handled well, can act as stepping-stones to greater mental fortitude and personal growth. It is often in the furnace of adversity that the steel of character is forged. Identifying learning experiences within pressure situations not only bolsters resilience but also fortifies a mental container, empowering you to navigate future high-pressure scenarios with greater ease and effectiveness.

10.5. Practical Strategies to Handle High-Pressure Situations

Next, we delve into tangible strategies that can be instrumental in weathering high-pressure situations with grace and grit. Beginning with preparatory measures, it's important to include stress conditioning exercises in your daily routine. These may involve putting oneself deliberately in taxing situations to build tolerance and resilience. It's also crucial to maintain a healthy lifestyle, as physical fitness significantly impacts mental endurance and stress management capabilities.

In the throes of high-pressure situations, it's essential to stay rooted in the present, employ effective decision-making strategies, and remain open to feedback. Creatively challenging your problem-solving skills keeps the mind flexible and adaptable, while feedback provides scope for improvement and precision.

Post-event reflection is an equally important part of handling high-pressure situations. Even seeming failures can contain valuable lessons; it's essential to recognize and utilize them for personal and professional growth.

Harnessing the warrior spirit means facing trials fearlessly, remaining resilient amidst chaos, and emerging victorious from high-pressure situations. With courage, perseverance, and the right strategies, pressure can indeed be turned into a tool of empowerment and excellence, creating not a crisis but an opportunity for growth and transformation. By integrating these strategies and shifting your perspective, you invite the possibility of becoming more confident, adaptable, stronger, and truly unshakeable.

Chapter 11. Living as A Warrior: Sustaining Unshakeable Confidence

Living as a warrior is a journey, an ongoing process of self-discovery, growth, and transformation. It is not a destination you arrive at but a path you walk, continuously generating that wealth of unshakeable confidence in every aspect of your life. The warrior life is a life of resilience, power, and courage; persistently battling fears and negativity, thriving amidst high-pressures, and bouncing back from challenges stronger every time. This chapter presents an extensive exploration of living as a warrior by sustaining unshakeable confidence.

11.1. What Does it Mean to Live as a Warrior?

Living as a warrior is about embracing you, the raw and pure you, aligning your thoughts, values, and actions with your true self. The warrior's existence can be likened to a single drop in an infinite ocean: it is a part of the whole, yet it carries within it the entirety of the ocean. Similarly, each of us has within us the strength, wisdom, and resilience of a warrior, waiting to be tapped.

Living as a warrior involves preserving your self-belief, nurturing your personal power, building steadfast resilience, and rising above fears and negativity. It's about embodying the warrior spirit, persisting in the face of adversity, and thriving under pressure.

11.2. Unshakeable Confidence: The Warrior's Badge

Unshakeable confidence lies at the core of the warrior's attitude. It is what drives them forward, keeps them standing in adversity, and fuels their journey of growth. This confidence isn't devoid of doubts or fears; it acknowledges them and overcomes them, converting every challenge into an opportunity for growth.

Unshakeable confidence ensures that you remain unswerving even when the path seems treacherous, never doubting your ability to rise above challenges.

11.3. Embodying the Warrior Spirit every day

Sustaining your warrior spirit every day requires digging deep and acknowledging every facet of your being, embodying an unflinching acceptance of your strengths and weaknesses, successes and failures, fears and aspirations.

Living as a warrior means embarking on a journey of self-discipline and conscious effort. From making mindful food choices to seeking physical strength through exercise, from practicing mental peace through meditation to cultivating emotional strength via relationships, every single day gives you myriad chances to channel your warrior spirit.

Embodying the warrior spirit also means having the courage to stand firm under pressure, making tough decisions and facing their outcomes, understanding that confidence isn't about going unscathed but about rising strong even after defeat.

11.4. Keeping Your Warrior Flame Alive

To sustain your warrior spirit, you need to intentionally nurture it. Much like a flame requires constant tending, so does a warrior's spirit.

Keep your flame alive by consistently challenging yourself, exposing yourself to new situations, and expanding your horizons. Seek out discomfort since growth lies outside your comfort zone.

Revisit your vision regularly, allow it to guide you, and trust that you are following the right path. When you firm up with confidence, you embody the resilience of your inner warrior, allowing it to guide you and empower you.

11.5. Living Your Truth: The Pinnacle of the Warrior Journey

In the end, living as a warrior is about living your truth. It means consistently standing tall in your strength, embracing your vulnerability, and sharing your authenticity with the world.

Every choice you make, every action you take, every word you speak should be in complete alignment with your deepest truth. This absolute alignment will be the source of your unshakeable confidence as you continue to live as the warrior you are destined to be.

To conclude, living as a warrior is an arduous but rewarding journey. It requires continual nurturing of self-belief, banishing self-doubt, embracing challenges, harnessing personal power, cultivating resilience, sustaining discipline, thriving under pressure, and above all, living your truth. It's not an easy path, but once embarked, you'll discover inner peace, strength, and unshakeable confidence that will forever fuel your journey to excellence.